I0706525

Table Of Contents

Chapter 1: Introduction to Age Regression Meditations for Little's

Understanding Age Regression Meditations

Age regression meditations are a powerful tool for little's who are struggling with sleep difficulties, self-esteem issues, and depression. These guided meditations can help you tap into your inner child and create a safe and comforting space where you can heal and find peace.

Age regression is a technique that allows you to reconnect with the younger version of yourself. It can be a way to explore and heal past traumas, release negative emotions, and cultivate self-love and acceptance. By immersing yourself in age regression meditations, you can create a nurturing environment where you can feel safe and supported.

For little's with sleep difficulties, age regression meditations can be especially helpful. They can help you relax your body and mind, release any tension or anxiety that may be keeping you awake, and guide you into a deep and restful sleep. These meditations often incorporate soothing music, gentle visualizations, and comforting affirmations to create a peaceful and calming atmosphere.

If you're struggling with self-esteem issues, age regression meditations can be a powerful tool for building self-confidence and self-worth. They can help you reconnect with the innocent and carefree aspects of your inner child, reminding you of your inherent value and worthiness. These meditations often focus on cultivating self-love, acceptance, and forgiveness, allowing you to let go of any negative self-perceptions and embrace your true self.

Additionally, age regression meditations can provide support for little's who are battling with depression. They can help you tap into the joy and wonder of childhood, reminding you of the simple pleasures in life. These meditations often incorporate playful imagery, joyful affirmations, and uplifting music to lift your spirits and bring a sense of lightness and happiness into your heart.

Remember, age regression meditations are a personal journey, and everyone's experience will be unique. It's essential to approach these meditations with an open mind and heart, allowing yourself to fully immerse in the experience. Be patient with yourself, as healing takes time, and trust the process.

In "Sweet Dreams: Age Regression Meditations for Little's with Sleep Difficulties," you will find a collection of guided meditations specifically designed to address the challenges faced by little's with sleep difficulties, self-esteem struggles, and depression. These meditations provide a safe and nurturing space for you to explore your inner child and find healing and comfort. Embrace the journey, and may sweet dreams await you.

Benefits of Age Regression Meditations for Little's

Benefits of Age Regression Meditations for Littles

Age Regression Meditations for Littles have proven to be a powerful tool for those facing sleep difficulties, self-esteem struggles, and depression. These guided meditations are specifically designed to help Littles find comfort, relaxation, and healing through age regression techniques.

One of the main benefits of age regression meditations is their ability to promote better sleep patterns. Littles often struggle with falling asleep or staying asleep due to anxiety or racing thoughts. By guiding Littles through a calming and soothing meditation, these techniques can help clear the mind, relax the body, and create a sense of security. This enables Littles to drift off into a restful sleep, waking up feeling refreshed and rejuvenated.

Moreover, age regression meditations can be highly beneficial for Littles struggling with self-esteem issues. These meditations provide a safe space for Littles to reconnect with their inner child, exploring and embracing their innocence, playfulness, and worthiness. By cultivating self-love and acceptance, Littles can develop a stronger sense of confidence and a positive self-image.

Furthermore, for Littles battling depression, age regression meditations offer a unique approach to healing. By tapping into the carefree and joyful aspects of childhood, these meditations can help Littles reconnect with their inner happiness and rediscover the beauty in life. The soothing and nurturing nature of these meditations can help alleviate symptoms of depression and create a sense of hope and optimism.

In addition to these specific benefits, age regression meditations can also provide a general sense of peace and tranquility. Littles who practice these meditations often report feeling a deep sense of relaxation, comfort, and safety. This can help reduce overall stress levels and promote emotional well-being.

If you are a Little struggling with sleep difficulties, self-esteem issues, or depression, age regression meditations can be a powerful tool to help you find peace and healing. By embracing your inner child, you can tap into a wellspring of strength, resilience, and joy. It is important to remember that you are worthy of love, care, and happiness, and age regression meditations can guide you on this journey of self-discovery and self-acceptance.

Sweet Dreams: Age Regression Meditations for Littles with Sleep Difficulties offers a collection of soothing and uplifting meditations tailored specifically for Littles. Whether you are seeking better sleep, improved self-esteem, or relief from depression, these age regression meditations can help you find solace, healing, and sweet dreams.

How to Use This Book

Welcome, Little's, to "Sweet Dreams: Age Regression Meditations for Little's with Sleep Difficulties." This book has been specially designed to help you relax, unwind, and overcome the challenges you may be facing in your sleep routine. Whether you are struggling with sleep difficulties, self-esteem issues, or even depression, these age regression meditations are here to support you.

Before we embark on this journey together, it is essential to understand how to make the most of this book. Here are some guidelines to help you get started:

1. Find a quiet and comfortable space: Choose a cozy corner in your room or any place where you feel safe and relaxed. Ensure that the environment is free from distractions so that you can fully immerse yourself in the meditations.

2. Set aside dedicated time: Make a commitment to yourself to devote some time each day to practice these meditations. Establishing a routine will help you experience the full benefits of the age regression techniques.

3. Follow the instructions: Each meditation is carefully crafted to guide you through a soothing and calming experience. Read the instructions carefully before starting and try to follow them as closely as possible. Remember, these meditations are tailored to address your specific needs.

4. Embrace your inner child: Age regression meditations encourage you to tap into your inner child. Let go of any inhibitions and allow yourself to fully engage with the meditations. Allow your imagination to soar and embrace the magical world of relaxation.

5. Practice self-care: Remember, this book is a tool to support your well-being. Alongside practicing the meditations, prioritize self-care in your daily routine. Engage in activities that bring you joy, spend time with loved ones, and seek support when needed. You deserve to be happy and cared for.

6. Reflect and journal: After each meditation, take a few moments to reflect on your experience. Consider jotting down your thoughts, feelings, and any insights you gained during the session. This will help you track your progress and understand the positive changes happening within you.

By following these guidelines, you will embark on a transformative journey towards better sleep, enhanced self-esteem, and a happier state of mind. Remember, "Sweet Dreams" is here to support you every step of the way.

So, dear Little's, get ready to embark on a magical adventure filled with soothing meditations, peaceful dreams, and a renewed sense of self. Let's dive in and create a bedtime routine that leads to sweet dreams and a brighter tomorrow.

Tips for a Successful Age Regression Meditation Practice

Age regression meditations can be a powerful tool for Little's who struggle with sleep difficulties, self-esteem issues, and depression. By tapping into your inner child and creating a safe and nurturing environment, these meditations can help you find comfort, healing, and a sense of peace. Here are some tips to make your age regression meditation practice more successful:

1. Create a Safe Space: Find a quiet and comfortable space where you won't be disturbed. Set up your meditation area with soft pillows, blankets, stuffed animals, or any other items that make you feel safe and secure. This will help you relax and create a nurturing environment for your inner child.

2. Set an Intention: Before beginning your meditation, set a clear intention for what you want to achieve. Whether it's improving sleep, boosting self-esteem, or alleviating depression, having a specific goal in mind will help you focus your energy and attention during the practice.

3. Visualize Your Inner Child: Imagine yourself as a younger version of yourself, the Little within you. Picture them with love, compassion, and care. Connect with their innocence, curiosity, and joy. This visualization will help you establish a stronger bond with your inner child and tap into their needs and desires.

4. Use Guided Meditations: Utilize guided age regression meditations specifically designed for Little's with sleep difficulties, self-esteem struggles, or depression. These meditations will guide you through the process, providing gentle prompts and visualizations to help you connect with your inner child and address their specific challenges.

5. Practice Regularly: Consistency is key when it comes to age regression meditation. Set aside dedicated time each day to engage in this practice. Over time, your mind and body will become more attuned to the process, making it easier to slip into a relaxed and receptive state.

6. Journaling: Keep a journal to document your experiences during and after each meditation session. Note any insights, emotions, or memories that arise. This will help you track your progress and gain a deeper understanding of your inner child's needs and healing journey.

Remember, age regression meditations are a form of self-care and healing. Be patient with yourself, and allow the process to unfold naturally. With regular practice and a compassionate attitude, you can create a nurturing space for your inner child and experience profound healing and transformation. Sweet dreams await you on this beautiful journey of age regression meditation.

Chapter 2: Age Regression Meditations for Little's with Sleep Difficulties

The Importance of Sleep for Little's

In this subchapter, we will explore the crucial role that sleep plays in the lives of Little's. Sleep is not only essential for physical health but also for emotional well-being and cognitive development. As Little's who may struggle with sleep difficulties, it is vital to understand why a good night's rest is so important and how it can positively impact various aspects of your life.

First and foremost, sleep is essential for your overall health. It allows your body to repair and rejuvenate itself, ensuring that you wake up feeling refreshed and ready to take on the day. Without adequate sleep, you may experience fatigue, lack of energy, and difficulty concentrating. This can hinder your ability to engage in activities you enjoy and affect your performance in school or other areas of life.

For Little's with sleep difficulties, it is crucial to establish a consistent bedtime routine that promotes relaxation and calmness. Age regression meditations specifically designed for Little's with sleep difficulties can be incredibly beneficial in helping you wind down and prepare for a restful night's sleep. These meditations provide a safe and soothing space for you to release any worries or anxieties that may be keeping you awake.

Additionally, sleep plays a significant role in your emotional well-being. Lack of sleep can contribute to mood swings, irritability, and increased stress levels. It can also exacerbate symptoms of depression and self-esteem struggles. By prioritizing quality sleep, you are taking a proactive step towards improving your emotional health and overall happiness.

Age regression meditations for Little's with self-esteem struggles and depression can help you cultivate a positive mindset and reinforce self-love and self-acceptance. These meditations guide you through affirmations and visualizations that promote feelings of worthiness and help you find inner peace.

Remember, sleep is not a luxury; it is a necessity. By understanding the importance of sleep and incorporating age regression meditations into your routine, you can improve your sleep patterns and enhance your overall well-being. Sweet dreams await you, Little's, so take the time to nurture yourself and create a peaceful bedtime routine that will help you drift off into a world of rest and tranquility.

Common Sleep Difficulties Faced by Little's

Sleep is an essential part of our daily lives, providing us with the rest and rejuvenation necessary to function at our best. However, for Little's who struggle with sleep difficulties, bedtime can quickly become a source of stress and frustration. In this subchapter, we will explore some of the common sleep difficulties faced by Little's and provide age regression meditations specifically designed to help overcome these challenges.

One of the most prevalent sleep difficulties Little's encounter is bedtime anxiety. The thoughts and worries that can plague their minds as they lie in bed can make it difficult for them to relax and fall asleep. Our age regression meditations for Little's with sleep difficulties address this issue by incorporating calming visualizations and soothing affirmations. Through guided imagery, Little's can imagine themselves in a safe and comforting environment, allowing their worries to melt away and promoting a sense of relaxation and serenity.

Another common sleep difficulty that Little's may experience is insomnia. Difficulty falling asleep or staying asleep throughout the night can leave them feeling tired and irritable during the day. Our age regression meditations for Little's with sleep difficulties aim to combat insomnia by incorporating mindfulness techniques and relaxation exercises. By focusing on their breath and allowing their bodies to gradually unwind, Little's can cultivate a state of deep relaxation that promotes better sleep.

Sleep difficulties can also be linked to self-esteem struggles and depression. Little's who struggle with low self-esteem or feelings of sadness may find it challenging to find peace and tranquility at bedtime. Our age regression meditations for Little's with self-esteem struggles and depression address these underlying issues by incorporating affirmations that promote self-love, acceptance, and positivity. By cultivating a sense of inner peace and confidence, Little's can create a more conducive environment for restful sleep.

In conclusion, this subchapter provides age regression meditations specifically tailored to address the common sleep difficulties faced by Little's. By incorporating calming visualizations, mindfulness techniques, and affirmations, these meditations aim to promote relaxation, overcome anxiety, combat insomnia, boost self-esteem, and alleviate symptoms of depression. Little's can embark on a journey towards sweet dreams and restful nights, allowing them to wake up feeling refreshed and ready to embrace the day ahead.

Creating a Calming Bedtime Routine

Bedtime can often be a challenging time for us little's, especially when we struggle with sleep difficulties, self-esteem struggles, or even depression. But fear not, my dear little's, for we have the power to create a calming bedtime routine that will help us drift off into sweet dreams.

The first step in creating a calming bedtime routine is to establish a consistent sleep schedule. Our little bodies thrive on routine, so try to go to bed and wake up at the same time every day. This will help regulate our internal clock and make it easier for us to fall asleep.

Once we have our sleep schedule in place, it's time to create a peaceful environment in our bedroom. Remove any distractions or stimulating items that may keep us awake, such as electronic devices or bright lights. Instead, fill our space with soft, cozy blankets and pillows that make us feel safe and secure.

Next, let's engage in relaxing activities before bed. This could include reading a comforting storybook, listening to soft music, or practicing age regression meditations specifically designed for little's with sleep difficulties. These meditations will guide us through a soothing journey, helping us let go of any worries or anxieties that may be keeping us awake.

After we have engaged in calming activities, it's important to practice self-care rituals that promote relaxation. This could involve taking a warm bath with lavender-scented bubbles or engaging in gentle stretching exercises. These rituals will not only help our bodies unwind but also send a signal to our minds that it's time to relax and prepare for sleep.

Finally, it's essential to cultivate a positive mindset before bed. For little's struggling with self-esteem or depression, this may require a little extra effort. Consider writing down three things we are grateful for or reciting positive affirmations that remind us of our worth and strength. By focusing on the positive, we can shift our mindset and create a more peaceful state of mind before drifting off to sleep.

Remember, my dear little's, creating a calming bedtime routine takes time and patience. But with consistency and dedication, we can transform our sleep experience and invite sweet dreams into our lives. So, tuck yourself in, close your eyes, and let the peaceful routine guide you into a restful slumber. Sleep tight, little ones!

Guided Meditation for Relaxation before Bed

Welcome to the subchapter on "Guided Meditation for Relaxation before Bed" from the book "Sweet Dreams: Age Regression Meditations for Little's with Sleep Difficulties." This section is specifically designed to help little's find calmness and tranquility before bedtime, allowing for a peaceful and restful night's sleep.

Bedtime can often be a challenging time for little's, especially those with sleep difficulties, self-esteem struggles, or depression. It is essential to create a bedtime routine that includes relaxation techniques to help calm the mind and prepare the body for sleep. Guided meditation is a powerful tool that can assist in achieving this state of deep relaxation.

In this subchapter, you will find a series of guided meditations tailored to your needs. These meditations will help little's let go of the day's worries and anxieties, allowing them to unwind and experience a sense of peace and tranquility. By incorporating these meditations into your bedtime routine, you will create a safe and comforting space that promotes a restful night's sleep.

The guided meditations in this subchapter will focus on various techniques such as deep breathing exercises, visualization, and positive affirmations. You will be guided to imagine yourself in a calm and serene environment, allowing your mind to wander and detach from any negative thoughts or emotions.

By practicing these meditations regularly, you will not only improve your sleep quality but also boost your self-esteem and alleviate symptoms of depression. The power of meditation lies in its ability to create a deep sense of relaxation and self-awareness, which can have profound effects on your overall well-being.

Remember, you are not alone in your struggles. Many little's face similar challenges, and by incorporating these age regression meditations into your daily routine, you are taking a proactive step towards improving your sleep and emotional well-being.

So, snuggle up in your cozy bed, close your eyes, and let the soothing words guide you into a state of deep relaxation. Sweet dreams await you as you embark on this journey of self-discovery and tranquility.

Note: It is always advisable to consult with a healthcare professional or therapist before incorporating any new practices into your routine, especially if you have underlying health conditions or concerns.

Guided Meditation for Falling Asleep Peacefully

In this subchapter, we will explore a guided meditation specifically designed to help Little's fall asleep peacefully. Sleep difficulties can be challenging, and we understand how important it is for you to have a good night's rest. This meditation aims to create a calm and soothing environment for your mind and body to relax, allowing you to drift off into a peaceful slumber.

Find a comfortable spot in your bed, snuggle up under your favorite blanket, and let's begin. Close your eyes and take a deep breath, inhaling positivity and exhaling any worries or stress. Imagine yourself in a beautiful meadow, surrounded by soft grass and colorful flowers. The warm sun rays gently caress your skin, filling you with a sense of tranquility.

As you continue to breathe deeply, imagine a gentle breeze sweeping over your body, carrying away any tension or anxious thoughts. Feel your body becoming lighter with each breath, sinking deeper into relaxation. Picture a cozy little cottage nestled at the edge of the meadow. This cottage is your safe haven, a place where you can truly be yourself.

Step inside and notice the warm glow of a crackling fireplace. The room is filled with soft pillows and stuffed animals, all there to provide you comfort and reassurance. Choose a cozy spot to curl up and make yourself at home. Close your eyes and imagine a gentle lullaby playing softly in the background, soothing your mind and body.

As you lay there, feel the weight of the day slowly lifting off your shoulders. Allow any negative thoughts or worries to dissolve, leaving space for peaceful and positive energy to flow through you. Visualize a soft, glowing light surrounding your body, cocooning you in a sense of security and love.

As you relax deeper into this meditation, imagine the meadow outside your cottage slowly fading away, replaced by a starry night sky. Each twinkling star represents a positive thought or affirmation. Choose one star and let it guide you into a deep and restful sleep. Visualize yourself floating among the stars, feeling safe and serene.

Know that you are loved, cherished, and deserving of a good night's sleep. Allow the comforting embrace of this guided meditation to guide you into dreamland, where worries are replaced by joy and tranquility. Feel yourself drifting off, knowing that you will awake refreshed and ready for a new day.

Remember, even on nights when sleep seems elusive, this guided meditation will always be here to guide you into a peaceful slumber. Sweet dreams, Little's. You are strong, resilient, and capable of overcoming any sleep difficulties that may come your way. Rest well, for tomorrow is a brand new adventure.

Morning Meditation for a Restful Night's Sleep

Welcome to the subchapter titled "Morning Meditation for a Restful Night's Sleep" from the book "Sweet Dreams: Age Regression Meditations for Little's with Sleep Difficulties." This subchapter is specifically designed for Little's who struggle with sleep difficulties, self-esteem struggles, and depression.

Mornings can be tough after a restless night's sleep. But fear not, for this morning meditation will help you start your day off on the right foot and set the stage for a restful night's sleep ahead.

Find a comfortable place to sit or lie down, closing your eyes gently. Take a deep breath in, filling your lungs with fresh air, and exhale slowly, releasing any tension in your body.

Imagine yourself in a peaceful garden, surrounded by beautiful flowers and gentle sunlight. Feel the warmth of the sun on your skin and the soft grass beneath your feet. As you walk through the garden, you come across a cozy little cottage.

Step inside and find a comfortable spot to sit or lie down. Take a moment to set an intention for your day, such as "I am calm and at peace" or "I am deserving of love and happiness." Repeat this intention silently to yourself a few times, allowing it to sink deep into your subconscious mind.

Now, visualize a glowing ball of light above your head. This ball of light represents all the positive energy and healing that you need for a restful night's sleep. See the light slowly descending towards you, enveloping your entire body in its warm embrace. Feel the light soothing your mind, body, and soul, releasing any worries or anxieties that may have kept you awake during the night.

Take a moment to express gratitude for this peaceful moment and for the opportunity to start your day with a fresh perspective. Visualize yourself going about your day with confidence and joy, knowing that you are deserving of love and happiness.

When you are ready, slowly open your eyes and bring your awareness back to the present moment. Carry the positive energy and intentions with you throughout your day, and trust that a restful night's sleep awaits you tonight.

Remember, you have the power to create a peaceful bedtime routine and conquer any sleep difficulties, self-esteem struggles, or depression you may be facing. Embrace this morning meditation as a tool to bring you closer to a restful night's sleep and a happier, healthier you.

Sweet dreams, Little's!

Diapered Sleep Sanctuary Guided Meditation

Welcome to the Diapered Sleep Sanctuary guided meditation, a special journey designed to help Little's with sleep difficulties find peace and comfort in their bedtime routine. Whether you struggle with falling asleep, staying asleep, or simply feeling safe and secure at night, this meditation is here to guide you towards a restful and rejuvenating sleep.

As you prepare for bedtime, find a cozy and comfortable spot where you can fully relax. Take a moment to adjust your diaper, ensuring it is snug and comforting, just like a warm hug. Take a deep breath in and exhale slowly, releasing any tension or worries from your day.

Close your eyes and imagine a magical sleep sanctuary, a place where you can feel completely safe and at ease. Picture a soft bed, adorned with fluffy pillows and cozy blankets, tailored just for you. Visualize the room filled with gentle, soothing colors and comforting scents, creating a peaceful atmosphere.

Now, envision a soft and glowing light radiating from above, enveloping you with a warm and loving energy. Allow this light to flow through every part of your body, from your head to your toes, bringing a sense of relaxation and calmness.

Imagine a soft lullaby playing in the background, its gentle melody soothing your soul. As you listen to the music, let your thoughts drift away, focusing only on the present moment. Feel the weight of the day lifting off your shoulders, leaving you feeling lighter and more at ease.

Now, let your mind wander to a happy memory or a place that brings you joy. It could be a favorite vacation spot, a cozy playroom filled with toys, or a peaceful garden surrounded by beautiful flowers. Take a moment to immerse yourself in this pleasant imagery, allowing it to fill you with happiness and peace.

As you begin to drift off to sleep, feel the gentle rhythm of your breath, slow and steady. Embrace the comforting sensation of your diaper, knowing that it keeps you safe and protected throughout the night. Allow yourself to surrender to the tranquility of sleep, knowing that tomorrow is a new day filled with endless possibilities.

Remember, dear Little, that you are loved and cherished. You deserve a peaceful and restful sleep, and this meditation is here to guide you towards that goal. May your dreams be sweet and your sleep be rejuvenating. Goodnight, little one.

Disclaimer: This meditation is not a substitute for professional medical advice. If you have any underlying medical conditions or concerns, please consult with a healthcare professional.

Guided Meditation Soft Sleepy Clouds

In this subchapter, we will explore the magical world of Guided Meditation Soft Sleepy Clouds, designed especially for little ones like you who are facing sleep difficulties. This meditation will help you drift off into a peaceful slumber, allowing you to experience the sweetest dreams.

Imagine yourself lying down on a cozy, fluffy cloud, surrounded by the softest and sleepiest clouds you have ever seen. These clouds are like companions, ready to carry you into a deep and restful sleep. As you settle in, take a deep breath in and slowly let it out, feeling all the tension in your body melt away.

Picture yourself gently floating on these clouds, as they carry you through the night sky. With each breath, you feel more relaxed, as if the clouds are wrapping you in a warm, comforting hug. As you continue to breathe deeply, you notice that the clouds change colors, creating a beautiful, calming atmosphere.

As you gaze up at the night sky, you see twinkling stars that seem to guide you towards a peaceful sleep. These stars represent all the positive thoughts and affirmations that will help you overcome any self-esteem struggles or feelings of sadness or depression.

Now, let's focus on your dreams. Imagine the clouds gently guiding you to a magical land where anything is possible. In this dreamland, you can be anything you want to be. You can fly like a bird, swim with dolphins, or even explore outer space. These dreams are filled with joy, happiness, and endless possibilities.

As you slowly drift off to sleep, know that you are safe and protected. The sleepy clouds will watch over you, keeping you calm and secure throughout the night. They will ensure that you have the most restful sleep, so you can wake up feeling refreshed and ready for a new day.

Remember, dear little one, this guided meditation is tailored just for you. It is designed to help you overcome sleep difficulties, boost your self-esteem, and ease any feelings of depression. Allow yourself to fully embrace this experience, knowing that you are deserving of a peaceful and restful sleep.

Close your eyes now and let the Guided Meditation Soft Sleepy Clouds carry you into a world of sweet dreams. May your slumber be filled with love, happiness, and tranquility.

Guided Meditation ABDL Diaper change

Subchapter: Guided Meditation ABDL Diaper Change

Welcome to the subchapter on Guided Meditation ABDL (Adult Baby Diaper Lover) Diaper Change. This specific meditation is designed to bring comfort, relaxation, and a sense of security to little ones who may struggle with sleep difficulties, self-esteem issues, or depression. By incorporating elements of age regression and focusing on the nurturing aspects of ABDL, this meditation aims to create a safe space for littles to find solace and healing.

In this meditation, you will be guided through a gentle visualization of a diaper change, allowing you to reconnect with your inner child and embrace your littleness. Find a quiet and comfortable place where you can relax and let go of any distractions. Take a few deep breaths, allowing your body and mind to unwind.

As the meditation begins, imagine yourself in a cozy nursery filled with soft toys, colorful walls, and a warm crib. Picture yourself lying on the changing table, wrapped in a soft blanket, surrounded by the loving presence of a caregiver. Feel their gentle touch as they begin to untape your wet diaper, removing it with care and attention.

Allow yourself to fully surrender to the experience, feeling the cool air on your skin as the caregiver cleanses and wipes you clean. Imagine the soothing sensation of a fresh diaper being placed beneath you and fastened securely, ensuring your comfort and protection.

As the diaper change concludes, feel a sense of relief and contentment washing over you. Embrace the feeling of being cared for and nurtured, knowing that you are safe and loved. Take a moment to notice the softness and warmth of the new diaper, reinforcing your sense of security.

Now, as you lie comfortably in your crib, allow yourself to drift off into a peaceful sleep. Feel the weight of the day lifting off your shoulders as you surrender to the gentle rhythm of your breath. Know that you are deserving of a good night's rest and that tomorrow is a new day filled with endless possibilities.

As you return to your waking state, carry the tranquility and love from this meditation with you. Remember that you can always revisit this visualization whenever you need a moment of comfort and reassurance.

May this Guided Meditation ABDL Diaper Change bring you the sweetest dreams and a renewed sense of self-esteem and happiness. You are cherished and deserving of all the love and care in the world. Sleep tight, little one.

Guided Meditation Bath time with Mummy

Bath time with Mummy is a special moment filled with warmth, comfort, and relaxation. In this guided meditation, you will embark on a journey to a magical world where bubbles and soothing water await you. As we go through this meditation, remember to breathe deeply and let your worries wash away.

Close your eyes and imagine yourself in a cozy bathroom with soft, fluffy towels and a warm, inviting bathtub. Mummy is by your side, ready to help you have the most relaxing bath time ever. She fills the tub with warm water, adding a few drops of your favorite lavender-scented bubble bath. As the water fills the tub, you feel a sense of calmness enveloping you.

Mummy gently helps you undress, and you step into the relaxing water. Feel the warmth embrace your body as you sink deeper into the tub. Close your eyes and imagine the water turning into a shimmering pool of light. This magical light soothes your mind and body, washing away any tension or worries you may have.

As you relax in the bath, Mummy starts pouring water over your head, gently massaging your scalp. Feel the water trickling down your face and neck, washing away any negative thoughts or emotions. With each pour, imagine the water cleansing your mind, leaving you feeling refreshed and renewed.

Now, imagine Mummy handing you a soft sponge. As you lather it with soap, feel the gentle touch against your skin. With each stroke, visualize the soap bubbles carrying away any stress or anxiety, leaving you feeling lighter and happier.

As the bath time comes to an end, Mummy helps you step out of the tub and wraps you in a fluffy towel. Feel the warmth and comfort of the towel as you snuggle into it. Mummy gently dries your body, making sure you feel cared for and loved.

Take a deep breath and slowly open your eyes, feeling rejuvenated and ready for a peaceful night's sleep. Remember, bath time with Mummy is not only about cleansing your body but also nurturing your soul. Embrace the love and comfort it brings, knowing that you are safe and cherished.

In this meditation, we have explored the power of bath time to wash away worries, boost self-esteem, and alleviate depression for little ones. By incorporating guided imagery, deep breathing, and visualization techniques, this meditation aims to create a safe and calming space for little's to unwind and find solace. Remember, you are not alone in your struggles, and there are always ways to find comfort and healing.

Diapered Dreamland Guided Meditation

Welcome to the magical world of Diapered Dreamland! This guided meditation is specially designed for Little's who are facing sleep difficulties, self-esteem struggles, or even depression. In this subchapter, we will embark on a journey to a place where all your worries and troubles melt away, and you can find comfort and peace.

As you settle down in a cozy and safe space, take a deep breath in and let it out slowly. Allow your body to relax, feeling the tension leaving your muscles. Imagine yourself snuggled up in your favorite soft blanket, feeling warm and secure.

Now, close your eyes and envision a beautiful, enchanted forest. The trees are tall and majestic, their leaves shimmering with a gentle breeze. As you enter this magical forest, you notice the soft sound of a babbling brook nearby. Follow the sound and let it guide you to a clearing in the woods.

In this clearing, you discover a sparkling waterfall cascading into a crystal-clear pool. The water is warm and inviting, like a giant bubble bath. Step into the pool and feel the warm water enveloping your body, washing away any negative thoughts or worries. As the water surrounds you, imagine it transforming into a soothing liquid, like a gentle hug from someone who loves you dearly.

As you relax in the pool, you notice a group of friendly woodland creatures gathering around you. They offer their support, love, and encouragement. These furry friends understand your struggles and want to help you feel better. Allow their comforting presence to soothe your heart and mind.

Now, it's time to float on a fluffy cloud towards Diapered Dreamland. With each gentle breeze, you feel lighter and more carefree. As you soar through the sky, you see cotton candy clouds and rainbows guiding your way. This is a place where dreams come true and happiness reigns supreme.

Finally, you land in Diapered Dreamland, a magical realm where your inner child can play, explore, and find joy. Here, you can embrace your true self and let go of any worries or doubts. Let the magic of this place fill your heart with happiness and contentment.

As you slowly return to your waking state, remember the feelings of peace and happiness you experienced in Diapered Dreamland. Carry this positivity with you throughout your day, knowing that you have the power to create your own little paradise, even in the real world.

You are loved, you are cherished, and you deserve all the happiness in the world. Sweet dreams, little one.

Chapter 3: Age Regression Meditations for Little's with Self-Esteem Struggles

Understanding Self-Esteem in Little's

Self-esteem is an essential aspect of our emotional well-being and plays a crucial role in our overall happiness and success in life. For Little's struggling with sleep difficulties, self-esteem issues can further exacerbate their challenges. In this subchapter, we will explore the concept of self-esteem in Little's, understanding its importance, and providing age regression meditations to help boost self-esteem and improve sleep patterns.

Self-esteem refers to how we perceive and value ourselves. It affects our thoughts, emotions, and behaviors, shaping our interactions with others and the world around us. For Little's, self-esteem struggles can manifest in various ways, such as feeling unworthy, lacking confidence, or constantly seeking validation from others. These challenges can lead to sleep difficulties and even depression.

Understanding the importance of self-esteem is the first step in addressing these issues. By recognizing that they are worthy, lovable, and deserving of love and care, Little's can start to shift their mindset and improve their overall well-being. It is crucial to remind Little's that their worth is not determined by external factors but lies within themselves.

Age regression meditations can be powerful tools in building self-esteem. Through guided visualization and affirmations, these meditations help Little's tap into their inner strength and develop a positive self-image. By revisiting past positive experiences or imagining future achievements, Little's can reframe negative thoughts and replace them with empowering beliefs. These meditations also provide a safe and nurturing space for Little's to heal emotional wounds and build resilience.

In addition to age regression meditations, it is essential to provide Little's with a supportive and loving environment. Encouraging open communication, validating their feelings, and celebrating their accomplishments can contribute to their self-esteem journey. Little's should be encouraged to engage in activities that bring them joy and help them discover their unique strengths and talents.

By addressing self-esteem struggles, Little's can experience improved sleep patterns and a sense of emotional well-being. As they cultivate self-love and acceptance, they will find it easier to relax, let go of anxieties, and drift into a peaceful sleep. Through the power of age regression meditations and a supportive environment, Little's can embark on a transformative journey towards greater self-esteem, happiness, and fulfillment.

Remember, Little's, you are special, loved, and deserving of all the happiness in the world. Embrace your uniqueness, believe in yourself, and let your self-esteem shine bright like a star in the night sky. Sweet dreams, little ones.

Identifying Signs of Low Self-Esteem in Little's

Identifying Signs of Low Self-Esteem in Littles

In the journey of age regression, it is essential to recognize and understand the signs of low self-esteem in Littles. Low self-esteem can hinder their emotional well-being, limit their potential, and impact their overall happiness. This subchapter aims to shed light on the signs of low self-esteem in Littles, helping them and their caregivers to identify and address these issues effectively.

1. Negative self-talk: Littles with low self-esteem often engage in negative self-talk, constantly criticizing themselves and undermining their abilities. They may use phrases like "I'm not good enough" or "I can't do anything right." Identifying these patterns of negative self-talk is crucial in helping Littles build a healthier self-perception.

2. Avoidance of challenges: Littles with low self-esteem may shy away from trying new things or taking on challenging tasks. They may fear failure and lack confidence in their abilities. Recognizing this avoidance behavior can help caregivers provide the necessary support and encouragement to help Littles overcome their self-doubt.

3. Seeking constant validation: Littles with low self-esteem often seek external validation to feel worthy or accepted. They may rely heavily on others' opinions and struggle to trust their own judgments. Encouraging Littles to develop self-validation techniques can enhance their self-esteem and reduce their dependence on external validation.

4. Social withdrawal: Littles with low self-esteem may isolate themselves from social interactions, feeling unworthy of others' company or fearing judgment. They may struggle with making friends, joining group activities, or expressing their opinions. Recognizing this social withdrawal is essential in providing a supportive and inclusive environment for Littles to flourish.

5. Perfectionism: Littles with low self-esteem often have high standards for themselves, striving for perfection in everything they do. They may become overly critical of their mistakes and feel inadequate when they don't meet their own unrealistic expectations. Acknowledging and helping Littles embrace their imperfections can foster self-acceptance and improve their self-esteem.

By identifying these signs of low self-esteem in Littles, caregivers and Littles themselves can take proactive steps to address these issues. Age regression meditations focusing on building self-esteem, self-acceptance, and self-love can be powerful tools in this journey. By providing a safe and nurturing environment, caregivers can help Littles develop a positive self-image, boost their confidence, and overcome the challenges that may arise from low self-esteem. Remember, every Little deserves to feel loved, valued, and confident in their own unique abilities.

Building a Positive Self-Image through Age Regression Meditations

In today's fast-paced and demanding world, it is easy for anyone, including little's, to develop self-esteem struggles and experience sleep difficulties or even depression. The constant pressure to meet societal expectations and the challenges of daily life can take a toll on our mental well-being. However, there is a powerful technique that can help little's overcome these obstacles and build a positive self-image: age regression meditations.

Age regression meditations for little's are a gentle and soothing way to tap into your inner child and heal any emotional wounds that may be causing sleep difficulties or self-esteem struggles. By revisiting and reconnecting with your younger self, you can rediscover the innocence, joy, and confidence that may have been lost along the way.

These meditations create a safe space where little's can explore their emotions, memories, and experiences in a comforting and nurturing environment. Through guided imagery and visualization, you will be able to address any negative beliefs or traumas that may be holding you back from embracing your true self. By gently releasing these limiting beliefs, you can begin to cultivate a positive self-image and develop a stronger sense of self-worth.

During age regression meditations, you will be guided to visualize yourself as a happy and carefree child. You will be encouraged to remember moments of joy, love, and accomplishment. By reliving these positive experiences, you can rewire your brain to focus on the positive aspects of yourself and your life, reducing the impact of negative thoughts and emotions.

These meditations also provide an opportunity to address any unresolved issues or traumas from your past. By revisiting these memories in a controlled and supportive environment, you can release any pent-up emotions and find healing and closure. This process allows you to let go of any self-doubt or negative self-perception that may have developed as a result of these experiences.

Through consistent practice of age regression meditations, little's can experience profound transformation. As you continue to connect with your inner child, you will develop a stronger sense of self-acceptance, self-love, and resilience. Sleep difficulties will gradually lessen as your mind becomes more at ease, leading to improved overall well-being.

If you are a little struggling with sleep difficulties, self-esteem struggles, or even depression, consider incorporating age regression meditations into your daily routine. These gentle and nurturing practices have the power to transform your self-image and bring back the sweet dreams you deserve. Embrace your inner child and unlock the path to a more positive and fulfilling life.

Guided Meditation for Boosting Self-Confidence

In this subchapter, we will delve into the world of guided meditation specifically designed to boost self-confidence. For our Little audience who may be struggling with sleep difficulties, self-esteem issues, or even depression, this meditation aims to uplift spirits, promote positive self-image, and provide a sense of inner strength.

Close your eyes and take a deep breath, feeling the warm air fill your lungs. As you exhale, let go of any negative thoughts or doubts that may be holding you back. Picture yourself in a serene and safe place, surrounded by beautiful colors and soothing sounds.

Now, imagine a gentle, loving voice guiding you through each step of this meditation. This voice encourages you to embrace your unique qualities and talents, reminding you that you are special and deserving of love and happiness.

As you continue to breathe deeply and relax, visualize a bright light above your head. This light represents your inner confidence. Let it slowly descend into your body, filling each and every cell with its radiant energy. Feel the warmth and power of this light as it spreads throughout your entire being.

Now, focus on your heart. Imagine a beautiful garden blooming with flowers. Each flower represents a positive trait or accomplishment that makes you proud. Take a moment to appreciate these qualities and achievements. Allow yourself to feel a deep sense of pride and self-acceptance.

Next, envision yourself in situations where you may typically feel anxious or self-conscious. See yourself confidently navigating these scenarios with ease and grace. Imagine the positive outcomes and the sense of accomplishment you will experience. Embrace the belief that you are capable of overcoming any obstacle and achieving your goals.

As the meditation comes to an end, take a moment to express gratitude for the newfound self-confidence you have cultivated. Remind yourself that this feeling of empowerment is always within reach, and you can return to this meditation whenever you need a boost.

Remember, dear Little, you are strong, resilient, and full of potential. With each meditation session, you are planting the seeds of self-confidence and nurturing them to grow into a beautiful garden of self-love and belief in your own abilities.

May this meditation guide you towards sweet dreams filled with self-assurance and a renewed sense of purpose. Sleep tight, Little one, knowing that you are loved and worthy of all the happiness in the world.

Guided Meditation for Self-Love and Acceptance

Subchapter: Guided Meditation for Self-Love and Acceptance

Welcome to the subchapter on guided meditation for self-love and acceptance. In this section, we will explore how age regression meditations can help little's who struggle with sleep difficulties, self-esteem issues, and depression to cultivate a sense of self-love and acceptance.

Being a little can sometimes be challenging, and it's important to remember that you are loved and cherished just as you are. This guided meditation will guide you to connect with your inner self, allowing you to embrace your unique qualities and develop a deep sense of self-love and acceptance.

Find a comfortable position, either sitting or lying down, and take a few deep breaths. Close your eyes and let go of any tension or worries you may be carrying. Imagine a safe and peaceful place where you can fully relax.

As you settle into this serene environment, visualize a soft, warm light surrounding you. This light represents love and acceptance, and it fills every part of your being. With each breath, feel this light expanding, spreading love and acceptance throughout your body.

Now, bring your attention to your heart. Imagine a gentle, soothing voice within you, guiding you towards self-love and acceptance. This voice reminds you of your worth, your uniqueness, and the beauty that resides within you.

Allow this voice to lead you on a journey of self-discovery. Visualize yourself as a young child, full of innocence, curiosity, and joy. Embrace that inner child and offer them love, understanding, and acceptance. Feel the warmth of this love radiating from your heart, healing any past wounds or self-doubt.

Now, take a moment to reflect on your positive qualities, talents, and accomplishments. Celebrate your strengths and acknowledge the progress you have made. Embrace all aspects of yourself, including the areas you may perceive as flaws or imperfections. Remember, they make you uniquely you.

As the meditation comes to an end, take a deep breath and feel the love and acceptance within you. Know that you are deserving of love, kindness, and happiness. Carry this sense of self-love and acceptance with you as you go about your day, knowing that you are enough just as you are.

Remember, self-love is a journey, and it takes time and practice. By incorporating this guided meditation into your daily routine, you can cultivate a deep sense of self-love and acceptance, leading to improved sleep, enhanced self-esteem, and a brighter outlook on life.

You are loved, little one, and you deserve all the love and acceptance in the world. Sweet dreams, and always remember to love yourself.

Growing Confidence Tree Guided Meditation

Welcome to the subchapter on the "Growing Confidence Tree Guided Meditation," specifically designed for Little's who may be struggling with sleep difficulties, self-esteem issues, or even depression. This meditation aims to help you nurture your inner strength and cultivate a strong foundation of confidence, allowing you to blossom and thrive like a beautiful tree.

Find a comfortable and quiet space where you can relax and let go of any worries or distractions. Take a moment to close your eyes and take a deep breath in, feeling the air filling your lungs, and exhaling slowly, releasing any tension or negativity. Allow your body to sink into a state of deep relaxation.

Imagine yourself in a peaceful forest, surrounded by tall, majestic trees. In the center of this forest stands a special tree, your very own Growing Confidence Tree. Picture it in your mind, noticing its strong trunk, branches reaching towards the sky, and vibrant green leaves.

Now, visualize yourself as a tiny seed planted at the base of this tree. As you look around, you notice the sun shining warmly on you, providing nourishment and energy for your growth. Feel the love and support of the universe embracing you, just as the earth supports the roots of the Growing Confidence Tree.

As you continue to imagine yourself as this tiny seed, feel the warmth and love radiating from your heart. Visualize this love flowing down into the earth, nurturing your roots, and allowing them to grow deeper and stronger. With each breath, feel your roots extending further, anchoring you firmly to the ground.

As time passes, you notice that your seed begins to sprout, pushing through the earth's surface and growing into a small sapling. With each passing day, you grow taller and stronger, just like the Growing Confidence Tree. Feel the energy and confidence flowing through your entire being.

Now, visualize yourself as a beautiful tree, standing tall and proud, with branches reaching towards the sky. Notice the strength and resilience in your trunk, and the vibrant leaves that represent your growing confidence. Feel the sense of empowerment and self-assurance filling your entire being.

Take a moment to bask in the beauty of your Growing Confidence Tree, knowing that you have the power to overcome any sleep difficulties, self-esteem struggles, or depression. Trust in yourself and the strength that lies within you.

When you are ready, slowly bring your awareness back to the present moment. Open your eyes and take a deep breath, feeling refreshed and renewed. Remember, you are a magnificent tree, capable of facing any challenge that comes your way.

May your Growing Confidence Tree continue to flourish, guiding you towards a life filled with joy, self-love, and happiness.

Mirror of Kindness Guided Meditation

Welcome to the Mirror of Kindness Guided Meditation, a powerful tool designed specifically for Little's who struggle with sleep difficulties, self-esteem struggles, and depression. This meditation is part of the book "Sweet Dreams: Age Regression Meditations for Little's with Sleep Difficulties," and it aims to provide a safe and nurturing space for you to explore and cultivate kindness within yourself.

Find a cozy and comfortable spot where you can relax and unwind. Take a moment to close your eyes and take a deep breath in, allowing any tension or worries to melt away. As you exhale, imagine yourself entering a magical room filled with mirrors.

In this room, you will find the Mirror of Kindness. Step closer and take a look at your reflection. Notice how you appear in the mirror. Do you see a Little who is tired, sad, or struggling? Allow yourself to acknowledge these feelings without judgment or criticism.

Now, imagine that the mirror starts to glow with a warm and gentle light. As the light envelops you, begin to see a transformation within yourself. Notice how your appearance changes, becoming brighter and happier. This is the reflection of your inner kindness and strength.

Take a moment to reflect on all the kind acts you have done for others, big or small. Allow these memories to fill you with warmth and joy. Feel the love and compassion you have shared with others, and let it radiate from within you.

Now, shift your focus to yourself. Look into the mirror and repeat the following affirmations:

"I am kind and deserving of love."

"I am worthy of happiness and peace."

"I am strong and capable of overcoming any challenges."

Take a few more moments to bask in the positive energy and self-love that the Mirror of Kindness has awakened within you. Feel the kindness flowing through your body and spreading to every cell, bringing healing and comfort.

When you are ready, slowly open your eyes and take a deep breath. Carry this newfound kindness and self-love with you throughout your day, knowing that you have the power to make a positive difference in your own life and the lives of others.

Remember, the Mirror of Kindness is always available to you whenever you need a gentle reminder of your own strength and resilience. Embrace the power of kindness and let it guide you towards sweet dreams and a brighter tomorrow.

May you always find comfort in the Mirror of Kindness.

Rainbow of Self-Love Guided Meditation

Subchapter: Rainbow of Self-Love Guided Meditation

Welcome to the magical world of age regression meditations, where you can embark on a journey of self-discovery and healing. In this subchapter, we will explore the "Rainbow of Self-Love" guided meditation, specifically designed for little ones just like you who may be struggling with sleep difficulties, self-esteem issues, or even depression.

Imagine yourself in a beautiful meadow, surrounded by vibrant flowers and gentle sunlight. Lie down on the soft grass and take a deep breath, feeling all your worries and stress begin to melt away. As you close your eyes, let your imagination take flight as we embark on a transformative adventure.

In this guided meditation, we will guide you through a rainbow of colors, each representing a different aspect of self-love. Imagine a vibrant red light surrounding your body, filling you with a sense of passion and strength. Feel the warmth radiating from this red light, reminding you of your inner power and resilience.

As we move on to the color orange, visualize it enveloping you in a warm embrace. This color represents joy and creativity. Allow yourself to tap into your playful side and embrace the wonders of your imagination.

Next, envision a bright yellow light bathing you in its glow. This color symbolizes self-worth and confidence. As the yellow light washes over you, feel a surge of self-assurance and belief in your abilities.

Now, picture a soothing green light enveloping your body, representing love and compassion. With each breath, allow this green light to fill your heart, reminding you of your capacity for kindness and empathy towards yourself and others.

Moving up the spectrum, imagine a calming blue light washing over you. This color represents peace and tranquility. Feel the soothing energy of the blue light releasing any tension or anxiety you may be feeling, allowing you to find serenity in the present moment.

Lastly, visualize a majestic purple light surrounding you, symbolizing wisdom and spirituality. As the purple light engulfs you, tap into your inner wisdom and connect with your higher self. Allow this light to guide you towards a deeper understanding of yourself and the world around you.

As the meditation comes to an end, slowly become aware of your surroundings, feeling a renewed sense of self-love and acceptance. Remember, you are a unique and special individual deserving of love and happiness. Embrace the power of this rainbow of self-love, carrying it with you into your waking life.

Sweet dreams, little one, as you continue your journey towards healing and self-discovery.

Affirmations for Daily Self-Esteem Improvement

In this subchapter, we will explore powerful affirmations that can help little ones with their daily self-esteem improvement. Affirmations are positive statements that can reshape our thoughts and beliefs, paving the way for self-love, confidence, and a healthy mindset. By practicing these affirmations regularly, you can gradually boost your self-esteem, overcome sleep difficulties, and find inner peace.

1. "I am loved and cherished just as I am."

Repeat this affirmation to remind yourself that you are worthy of love and acceptance. Embrace your unique qualities and understand that you are valuable just the way you are.

2. "I am brave and capable of facing any challenge."

Use this affirmation to build confidence and courage. Believe in your abilities to overcome obstacles and tackle any situation that comes your way.

3. "I deserve happiness, and I choose to be joyful every day."

Remind yourself that happiness is your birthright. By affirming your right to joy, you invite positivity and happiness into your life.

4. "I am surrounded by people who support and uplift me."

Affirm that you have a strong support system. Visualize yourself surrounded by loving friends, family, and caregivers who offer encouragement and believe in your potential.

5. "I am enough, and my worth is not defined by external factors."

Acknowledge that your worth is intrinsic and not dependent on external validation or achievements. You are enough just by being yourself.

6. "I am resilient, and I can overcome any challenge."

Reinforce your resilience by affirming your ability to bounce back from setbacks. Believe in your strength and know that you have the power to overcome any difficulty.

7. "I am worthy of love and kindness."

Affirm your deservingness of love, care, and kindness. Treat yourself with compassion and extend the same kindness to others.

Remember to practice these affirmations daily, ideally during your bedtime routine. Allow their positive energy to seep into your subconscious mind, helping you to overcome sleep difficulties, self-esteem struggles, and depression. By embracing these affirmations, you can transform your mindset and create a nurturing environment for your emotional well-being.

Note: It is crucial to consult with a mental health professional for severe sleep difficulties, self-esteem struggles, or depression. This book aims to provide additional support and complement professional guidance.

Cuddly Confidence Blanket Guided Meditation

Welcome to the subchapter titled "Cuddly Confidence Blanket Guided Meditation" from the book "Sweet Dreams: Age Regression Meditations for Little's with Sleep Difficulties." This chapter is specifically designed for Little's who may be struggling with sleep difficulties, self-esteem issues, or even depression. Through this guided meditation, we aim to provide comfort, confidence, and a sense of security to help you have a peaceful and restful sleep.

As you settle into your cozy bed, imagine yourself wrapped up in a soft, cuddly blanket. This special blanket is infused with love, warmth, and positivity. It is your confidence blanket, here to protect and support you throughout this meditation.

Take a deep breath in and let it out slowly. Allow any tension or worries to fade away with each exhale. As you continue to breathe deeply, imagine a warm, golden light surrounding your body, gently embracing you like a cozy hug.

Now, imagine that the blanket is magically transforming into a beautiful garden, filled with vibrant flowers and gentle butterflies. Each flower represents a unique quality that makes you special and loved. Take a moment to visualize these flowers in your mind's eye, noticing their colors, shapes, and fragrances.

As you explore this magical garden, you come across a mirror. Look into the mirror and see yourself, wearing a big smile and radiating confidence. Affirm to yourself, "I am loved, I am worthy, and I am enough." Repeat this affirmation several times, allowing it to sink deep into your heart.

Now, imagine the butterflies gently landing on your shoulders, whispering words of encouragement and love. Feel their delicate touch, filling you with a renewed sense of self-esteem and positivity. Allow their whispers to uplift your spirit and fill your mind with happy thoughts.

As you start to feel more relaxed and at peace, imagine yourself curling up under the blanket once again. Let it wrap around you, providing warmth, comfort, and a sense of security. Feel the love and support of the blanket, knowing that it will always be there for you, even when you're not meditating.

Take a few more deep breaths, feeling the calmness and tranquility washing over you. When you're ready, slowly open your eyes, carrying the confidence and peace from this meditation into your day or night.

Remember, you are worthy, loved, and capable of achieving anything you set your mind to. Embrace your inner strength and let your confidence shine through like a bright star in the sky.

Sweet dreams, dear Little's. May your sleep be peaceful and your heart be filled with confidence and joy.

Chapter 4: Age Regression Meditations for Little's with Depression

Understanding Depression in Little's

Understanding Depression in Littles

Depression is a complex and challenging condition that can affect individuals of all ages, including little's. It is important for little's and their caregivers to have a clear understanding of depression, its causes, symptoms, and available treatments. This subchapter aims to provide a comprehensive understanding of depression in littles, helping them navigate through their emotions and find ways to cope with their struggles.

Depression in littles may manifest differently compared to adults. Littles may exhibit symptoms such as persistent sadness, irritability, loss of interest in activities they once enjoyed, changes in appetite and sleep patterns, low energy levels, difficulty concentrating, and feelings of worthlessness. It is crucial for caregivers to recognize these signs and offer support to their little one.

Understanding the underlying causes of depression in littles is essential for effective management. Depression can be triggered by a range of factors, including trauma, loss, changes in routine or environment, social difficulties, or even genetics. By identifying such triggers, caregivers can work towards creating a safe and nurturing environment for their little to heal and flourish.

Age regression meditations can be a powerful tool in helping littles with depression. These meditations provide a safe space for littles to explore their emotions and release any negative feelings or thoughts. By guiding littles through relaxation techniques and gentle visualizations, age regression meditations can help them regain a sense of peace, security, and self-confidence.

In addition to age regression meditations, it is essential for littles with depression to receive professional help. Caregivers should consider consulting with a mental health professional who specializes in working with children and adolescents. Therapy sessions, such as play therapy or cognitive-behavioral therapy, can aid littles in understanding and managing their emotions, developing healthy coping strategies, and building resilience.

Remember, depression is not a sign of weakness or a character flaw. It is a medical condition that can be treated with the right support and interventions. By providing a nurturing and understanding environment, along with age regression meditations and professional help, littles with depression can find their way towards healing and enjoying a fulfilling childhood.

Note: The term "littles" refers to individuals who identify as having an age regression or littlespace within the BDSM community. This content should be approached within that context.

Recognizing Symptoms of Depression in Little's

Recognizing Symptoms of Depression in Littles

Depression is a complex and challenging condition that can affect individuals of all ages, including Littles. As a Little, it is important to understand the symptoms of depression so that you can seek the support and care you deserve. This subchapter aims to help you recognize the signs of depression and provide guidance on how to cope with these feelings.

For Littles, depression can manifest in various ways, often differing from how it appears in adults. Some common symptoms include persistent sadness or tearfulness, a loss of interest in activities you once enjoyed, changes in

appetite or sleep patterns, difficulty concentrating, and feelings of
worthlessness or guilt. It is crucial to remember that these symptoms can vary
from person to person, and it's essential to consult a mental health professional
for an accurate diagnosis.

If you find yourself experiencing these symptoms, it's crucial to reach out for
support. Talk to a caregiver, trusted friend, or family member who can help
you navigate these feelings. Remember, you are not alone, and there are
people who care about your well-being.

In addition to seeking support from those around you, incorporating age
regression meditations into your routine can be beneficial. Age regression
meditations for Littles with depression focus on promoting relaxation, self-
compassion, and positive affirmations. These meditations can help alleviate
some of the symptoms associated with depression, such as negative self-talk
and feelings of worthlessness.

During your meditation practice, visualize yourself in a safe and comforting
space, surrounded by your favorite toys and caregivers who love and support
you unconditionally. Engage your senses by imagining the smells, sounds, and
textures that bring you joy. Allow yourself to embrace the innocence and
playfulness that comes naturally to Littles, nurturing your inner child.

Remember, depression is a treatable condition, and seeking professional help
is crucial for your well-being. While age regression meditations can provide
temporary relief, they should not replace therapy or medical intervention.
Work closely with a mental health professional to develop a comprehensive
treatment plan that is tailored to your unique needs.

By recognizing the symptoms of depression and seeking support, you are
taking an important step toward healing and finding relief from your struggles.
Remember, you are strong, resilient, and deserving of happiness.

Promoting Emotional Well-being through Age Regression Meditations

In the journey of life, emotional well-being plays a crucial role in our overall happiness and fulfillment. For Little's who may be struggling with sleep difficulties, self-esteem issues, or even depression, age regression meditations can be a powerful tool to promote emotional well-being and bring about a sense of peace and tranquility.

Age regression meditations are a form of guided meditation that takes you back to a time when you were younger, allowing you to tap into your inner child and address any emotional challenges that may be hindering your present well-being. These meditations create a safe and nurturing space where Little's can explore their emotions, heal past wounds, and build a strong foundation for a brighter future.

For Little's with sleep difficulties, age regression meditations can help create a soothing bedtime routine that promotes relaxation and peaceful slumber. By revisiting pleasant memories and creating new positive experiences through visualization, these meditations can help calm anxious thoughts and invite a restful night's sleep.

Self-esteem struggles can often plague Little's, impacting their confidence and self-worth. Age regression meditations provide an opportunity to reconnect with the innocent and joyful aspects of childhood, where self-acceptance and love were abundant. By revisiting these moments, Little's can reawaken their sense of self-worth and cultivate a positive self-image, building a strong foundation for healthy self-esteem.

Depression can be a heavy burden to bear, but age regression meditations can offer solace and healing. By revisiting moments of joy, love, and positivity, these meditations can help lift the weight of depression and bring about a sense of hope and happiness. These guided journeys can create a safe haven for Little's, allowing them to process their emotions and find comfort in the healing power of their inner child.

In "Sweet Dreams: Age Regression Meditations for Little's with Sleep Difficulties," you will find a collection of guided meditations specifically designed to address the unique challenges faced by Little's. Each meditation is tailored to promote emotional well-being, whether it be improving sleep, boosting self-esteem, or alleviating depression. Through the power of age regression, you can rediscover your inner strength and resilience, paving the way for a more fulfilling and joyful life.

Remember, you are not alone in your struggles. With age regression meditations, you can find comfort, healing, and a renewed sense of well-being. Take this journey to reconnect with your inner child and embrace the sweet dreams that await you.

Guided Meditation for Finding Inner Peace and Happiness

In this subchapter, we will explore the power of guided meditation as a tool to help Little's find inner peace and happiness. Whether you are struggling with sleep difficulties, self-esteem issues, or depression, this guided meditation practice is designed to provide comfort and support on your journey to emotional well-being.

Close your eyes and take a deep breath. Imagine yourself in a peaceful and serene place, surrounded by beautiful colors and calming sounds. As you breathe in, feel the positive energy entering your body, and as you exhale, let go of any tension or negativity.

Now, picture a gentle, loving presence beside you. This presence is your guide, someone who understands your struggles and wants to help you find peace and happiness. Allow yourself to feel their love and support, knowing that you are not alone.

Together, you and your guide will embark on a journey within. As you travel through your mind, visualize any worries or anxieties as clouds in the sky. Watch as these clouds slowly dissolve and disappear, leaving behind a clear, blue sky.

Now, focus on your heart. Feel the warmth and love residing within. This is your inner peace. With each breath, allow this peace to expand, spreading throughout your entire body. Feel it filling every cell, soothing and calming any negative emotions.

As you continue to breathe deeply, imagine yourself surrounded by a golden light. This light represents pure happiness. Feel its warmth touching your skin and permeating your entire being. Allow this happiness to radiate from within you, filling your heart with joy.

Now, take a moment to reflect on the positive qualities within yourself. Think about the things you are good at, the things that make you special. Embrace these qualities and let them empower you. Remember, you are unique and deserving of love and happiness.

As the meditation comes to an end, take a moment to express gratitude for this experience and for the love and support you have received. Open your eyes and carry this inner peace and happiness with you throughout your day.

Remember, dear Little's, finding inner peace and happiness is a journey, and guided meditation can be a valuable tool to support you along the way. Allow yourself to embrace the love and guidance offered in this practice, and trust that you have the strength within you to find the peace and happiness you deserve.

Guided Meditation for Coping with Sadness and Grief

Subchapter: Guided Meditation for Coping with Sadness and Grief

Introduction:
In times of sadness and grief, it can be challenging for little ones to understand
and cope with their emotions. This guided meditation is designed to provide
comfort and support to those who are experiencing these difficult emotions.
By embracing age regression techniques, we aim to help little ones navigate
sadness and grief in a safe and gentle manner.

Meditation Script:
Find a cozy and quiet space where you can relax and let go of any worries.
Close your eyes and take a deep breath in, allowing your body to relax with
each exhale. Imagine yourself in a peaceful meadow, surrounded by soothing
colors and comforting sounds.

Visualize a gentle, loving presence beside you, someone you trust and feel safe
with. This could be a favorite stuffed animal or a caring imaginary friend. Feel
their warm embrace and know that they are here to support you through your
sadness and grief.

Acknowledge your emotions:
Take a moment to recognize and accept the sadness and grief you are
experiencing. It's okay to feel these emotions, and it's important to give
yourself permission to process them. Imagine the sadness as a soft, gray cloud
hovering above you. With each breath, visualize this cloud slowly dissipating,
allowing you to release the weight of your emotions.

Comfort through visualization:
Picture a beautiful, healing light surrounding you, radiating warmth and love.
This light is filled with positive energy and is here to bring you comfort.
Allow it to wrap around you like a cozy blanket, soothing your heart and soul.

Now, imagine a serene waterfall appearing before you. This waterfall is
infused with healing energy, and as you step into its gentle cascade, feel the
sadness and grief being washed away. The water cleanses your emotions,
leaving you feeling lighter and more at peace.

Self-compassion:

Repeat affirmations to yourself, such as "I am loved," "I am strong," and "I am deserving of happiness." Remind yourself that it's okay to grieve and that you are never alone in your journey. Picture a garden growing within your heart, filled with beautiful flowers representing self-love, strength, and resilience.

Conclusion:

As you slowly bring your awareness back to the present moment, take a moment to thank yourself for giving time and space to honor your emotions. Remember that the process of healing takes time, and it's important to be patient and gentle with yourself. Whenever you feel overwhelmed by sadness and grief, come back to this guided meditation to find solace and comfort. You are not alone, and there is always love and support available to you.

Sunrise of Renewal Guided Meditation

Welcome to the subchapter titled "Sunrise of Renewal Guided Meditation" from our book, "Sweet Dreams: Age Regression Meditations for Little's with Sleep Difficulties." In this chapter, we will explore a gentle and calming meditation practice designed specifically for little's who may be facing sleep difficulties, self-esteem struggles, or even depression.

The Sunrise of Renewal Guided Meditation is a powerful tool that will help you find solace, peace, and renewal within yourself. Just like the dawn of a new day, this meditation will guide you towards a fresh start, helping you let go of negative thoughts and emotions, and embrace a sense of rejuvenation.

Find a comfortable and quiet space where you can relax without any distractions. Close your eyes and take a deep breath, allowing your body to relax with each exhale. As you continue to breathe deeply, imagine yourself standing on a beautiful beach, feeling the warm sand beneath your toes and the gentle breeze caressing your face.

As the meditation progresses, visualize the sky slowly transitioning from darkness to a soft glow. The first rays of sunlight appear on the horizon, painting the sky with hues of gold, pink, and orange. Feel the warmth of the sun's rays on your skin, filling you with a sense of hope and renewal.

Allow yourself to be fully present in this moment, embracing the beauty and tranquility of the sunrise. As the sun continues to rise, imagine it melting away any negative thoughts, fears, or worries that may be weighing you down. With each ray of sunlight, feel your self-esteem growing stronger, your sleep becoming deeper and more restful, and your depression lifting, making room for happiness and joy.

As the meditation comes to a close, take a moment to express gratitude for this new beginning. Open your eyes slowly and carry this feeling of renewal with you throughout the day, allowing it to guide you towards a peaceful and positive mindset.

Remember, you are strong, resilient, and deserving of a fresh start. The Sunrise of Renewal Guided Meditation is here to support you on your journey towards a restful sleep, improved self-esteem, and a brighter outlook on life. Embrace this opportunity for renewal and watch as it transforms your life, one sunrise at a time.

Sweet dreams, little one.

Guided Meditation Joyful Inner Playground

Guided Meditation: Joyful Inner Playground

In this subchapter, we will explore a delightful and enchanting guided meditation called "Joyful Inner Playground." Designed specifically for little ones with sleep difficulties, self-esteem struggles, and even those battling with depression, this meditation aims to transport you to a world of immense joy, happiness, and wonder.

Close your eyes, take a deep breath, and imagine yourself standing in front of a magical gate. This gate is the entrance to your very own inner playground, a place where all your dreams come true. As you step through the gate, you find yourself surrounded by a vibrant, colorful landscape filled with joyous scenes and friendly creatures.

In this inner playground, you have the power to create and explore anything you desire. Picture yourself swinging high in the sky on a golden swing, feeling a sense of liberation and freedom. As you swing, notice how the wind gently brushes against your skin, carrying away any worries or negative thoughts.

Next, imagine a beautiful meadow filled with flowers of every color. Lay down on the soft grass and watch as fluffy clouds pass by in the sky above. Feel a sense of tranquility and peace wash over you, soothing any anxiety or sadness you may be feeling.

As you continue to explore this magnificent playground, you stumble upon a crystal-clear lake. Dip your toes into the water and notice how it sparkles like diamonds in the sunlight. Feel the coolness of the water and let it wash away any self-doubt or insecurities you may have.

In the distance, you see a magnificent castle standing tall. This castle represents your inner strength and resilience. Walk towards it with confidence, knowing that you are capable of overcoming any challenge that comes your way. As you enter the castle, feel a surge of empowerment and a renewed sense of self-worth.

Take a moment to reflect on the joy and happiness you have experienced in this inner playground. Know that this magical place is always within you, ready to be accessed whenever you need it. As you open your eyes, carry this sense of joy and empowerment with you into the world, knowing that you are strong, capable, and deserving of happiness.

Remember, dear ones, you have the power to create your own joyful inner playground. Embrace the magic within and allow it to guide you towards a peaceful night's sleep, enhanced self-esteem, and a renewed sense of hope. Sweet dreams, little ones.

Note: This content is intended for a niche audience of "Little's" who are seeking age regression meditations, particularly those with sleep difficulties, self-esteem struggles, and depression. It aims to provide a comforting and empowering experience through a guided meditation called "Joyful Inner Playground."

Guided Meditation Heartbeat of Hope

Subchapter: Guided Meditation - Heartbeat of Hope

Welcome, dear Little's, to the enchanting world of age regression meditations. Within the realms of your imagination, we shall embark on a journey of healing and discovery. This subchapter, titled "Heartbeat of Hope," is designed to help you find solace and strength, especially if you are facing sleep difficulties, struggling with self-esteem, or battling depression.

As you settle down in a cozy space, take a deep breath and let your worries float away. Close your eyes and imagine a gentle, warm light surrounding you, filling you with comfort and security. This light represents your inner strength and resilience.

Now, let us focus on your heartbeat. Feel the rhythmic pulsations resonating through your entire body. As you become aware of your heartbeat, imagine it transforming into a beacon of hope. Visualize this radiant light flowing from your heart, spreading throughout your entire being.

With each beat, you feel a surge of positivity and renewal. This heartbeat of hope reminds you that even in the darkest of times, there is always a glimmer of light. It reassures you that you are not alone, and there are people who care deeply about your well-being.

As the meditation continues, imagine yourself surrounded by a lush forest. The trees stand tall and strong, just like you. Their branches reach out, forming a protective canopy overhead. You can sense their wisdom and ancient presence.

Take a moment to breathe in the fresh forest air. With each inhalation, imagine your heart expanding with love and acceptance. Feel any negative thoughts or emotions being replaced by a sense of peace and self-worth. As you exhale, release any tension or self-doubt that may have weighed you down.

As you walk through this magical forest, you come across a sparkling river. Stand by its banks and dip your hand into the water. Feel its coolness and purity. This river represents the flow of life, constantly renewing and replenishing.

Imagine your heartbeat merging with the gentle rhythm of the river. As the water flows, it washes away any lingering sadness or negativity. Trust in the river's ability to cleanse your spirit and nourish your soul, leaving you refreshed and rejuvenated.

Before concluding this meditation, take a moment to express gratitude for your heartbeat of hope. Feel its warmth and energy infusing every aspect of your being. Know that you are capable of overcoming any challenge that comes your way.

When you are ready, gently open your eyes and return to the present moment, carrying the heartbeat of hope within you. Remember, dear Little's, you are never alone, and there is always hope waiting to guide you through the darkest nights into a brighter tomorrow.

Healing Balloon Release Guided Meditation

Subchapter: Healing Balloon Release Guided Meditation

Welcome to the healing balloon release guided meditation, a powerful tool to help you find peace and relaxation in your sleep. This meditation is specifically designed for Little's who struggle with sleep difficulties, self-esteem struggles, and depression. By tapping into the therapeutic benefits of age regression meditations, we will embark on a journey of healing and self-discovery.

Before we begin, find a comfortable place to sit or lie down. Take a deep breath in, and as you exhale, let go of any tension or worries that may be weighing you down. Allow your body to sink into the surface beneath you, feeling supported and safe.

Now, imagine yourself in a beautiful meadow surrounded by vibrant flowers and gentle breezes. Visualize a colorful balloon in front of you, representing all the negative emotions and thoughts you want to release. Take a moment to acknowledge these feelings, giving them space to be recognized.

Next, take a deep breath in, filling your lungs with fresh air, and as you exhale, imagine blowing all those negative emotions into the balloon. Visualize them transforming into wisps of smoke, leaving your body and mind. See the balloon expanding with each breath, becoming lighter and lighter.

As you continue to release your negative emotions, notice how your body feels lighter, your mind clearer, and your heart more at ease. The weight of these burdens is being lifted, allowing you to find a sense of calm and tranquility.

Now, gently tie a string to the balloon, symbolizing your intention to let go of these negative emotions. As you prepare to release the balloon, feel a sense of joy and freedom building within you. Take one final deep breath, and on the exhale, let go of the balloon, watching it float higher and higher into the sky.

As the balloon disappears from sight, imagine all the negative emotions dissipating into the vastness of the universe. Feel a renewed sense of lightness and peace within you, knowing that you have released what no longer serves you.

Take a moment to reflect on how this experience has brought you closer to a state of healing and self-acceptance. Embrace the positive affirmations that arise from this meditation, reminding yourself of your worth, strength, and the endless possibilities that lie ahead.

When you are ready, slowly bring your awareness back to the present moment. Take a few deep breaths, feeling the sensation of your body on the surface beneath you. Open your eyes and carry the sense of peace and rejuvenation with you as you continue on your journey of self-discovery and growth.

Remember, you have the power to heal and overcome any challenges you may face. Embrace the healing balloon release guided meditation as a tool to find solace, strength, and sweet dreams in your life.

Daily Rituals for Managing Depression

Managing depression can be challenging, but with the right daily rituals, you can take control of your emotions and find peace within yourself. In this subchapter, we will explore some powerful daily rituals specifically designed for "Little's" who are struggling with depression.

1. Morning Affirmations: Start your day by reciting positive affirmations that resonate with you. Affirmations like "I am loved," "I am worthy," and "I am strong" can help shift your mindset and set a positive tone for the day ahead.

2. Mindful Breathing: Throughout the day, take a few moments to focus on your breath. Close your eyes, take deep breaths, and imagine inhaling positivity and exhaling negativity. This simple practice can help calm your mind and ease depressive thoughts.

3. Gratitude Journaling: Before going to bed, write down three things you are grateful for each day. Focusing on the positives in your life can help shift your perspective and foster a sense of gratitude, which is crucial for managing depression.

4. Creative Expression: Engaging in creative activities such as drawing, coloring, or writing can be incredibly therapeutic. Allow yourself to explore your emotions through art, and use it as a form of self-expression and release.

5. Self-Care Routine: Develop a self-care routine that incorporates activities that bring you joy and comfort. Whether it's taking a warm bath, reading a favorite book, or cuddling with a stuffed animal, prioritize self-care activities that nourish your soul.

6. Emotional Release: Find healthy outlets to release your emotions, such as talking to a trusted friend, writing in a journal, or participating in age regression meditations specifically designed for managing depression. These meditations can help you explore your emotions and find healing.

7. Mindful Movement: Incorporate gentle exercises like stretching or yoga into your daily routine. Physical activity releases endorphins, which can elevate your mood and reduce symptoms of depression.

Remember, managing depression is a journey, and it's essential to be patient and kind to yourself along the way. By implementing these daily rituals, you can gradually create a positive shift in your mindset and find solace in your age regression journey.

Chapter 5: Conclusion

Recap of the Benefits of Age Regression Meditations for Little's

In the previous chapters, we have explored the wonderful world of age regression meditations and how they can positively impact the lives of Little's with sleep difficulties, self-esteem struggles, and depression. Now, let's recap the incredible benefits these meditations can bring to your life.

First and foremost, age regression meditations are a powerful tool for improving sleep patterns. By guiding you through a journey back to your younger self, these meditations create a safe and nurturing environment where you can let go of the worries and stressors of adulthood. As you reconnect with the innocence and joy of being a Little, you will find it easier to relax and drift off into a peaceful sleep.

Moreover, age regression meditations can work wonders for Little's struggling with self-esteem issues. Through these guided journeys, you will be able to rediscover your inner strength, resilience, and worthiness. By connecting with your younger self, you will remember how loved, cherished, and valued you were, and still are. This profound realization can help boost your self-esteem and bring about a sense of self-acceptance and confidence in your present life.

Furthermore, age regression meditations offer solace and healing for Little's dealing with depression. By revisiting the carefree and joyful moments of your childhood, you can tap into a wellspring of happiness and contentment. These meditations allow you to temporarily escape the weight of depression, providing you with a respite from negative thoughts and emotions. With regular practice, age regression meditations can even help rewire your brain, fostering a more positive mindset and a greater sense of emotional well-being.

In conclusion, age regression meditations have proven to be an invaluable tool for Little's with sleep difficulties, self-esteem struggles, and depression. By immersing yourself in these guided journeys, you can experience the countless benefits they bring, including improved sleep, enhanced self-esteem, and a greater sense of happiness and contentment. So, embrace the power of age regression meditations and let them guide you on a transformative journey towards a more fulfilling and peaceful life. Sweet dreams, Little's!

Encouragement for Continued Practice and Growth

In this subchapter, we want to address the importance of continued practice and growth for all the Little's out there who are facing sleep difficulties, self-esteem struggles, and depression. We understand that these challenges can be overwhelming, but we believe that with dedication and perseverance, you can find peace and happiness within yourself.

First and foremost, it's crucial to recognize that age regression meditations are a powerful tool for your well-being. They provide a safe space where you can explore your emotions, release any negative thoughts, and build a strong foundation for personal growth. By engaging in these meditations regularly, you are actively investing in your own healing and happiness.

Remember, progress takes time. Healing is not an overnight process, and it's essential to be patient with yourself. Some days may be more difficult than others, but even the smallest steps forward are significant achievements. Celebrate your successes, no matter how small they may seem, and be gentle with yourself when you face setbacks. This journey is about progress, not perfection.

Surround yourself with a supportive community. Seek out others who are also practicing age regression meditations and share your experiences with them. Connect with people who understand your struggles and can offer guidance and encouragement. Remember, you are not alone in this journey, and together, we can uplift one another.

Additionally, embrace self-care practices beyond meditation. Engage in activities that bring you joy and promote relaxation. Whether it's reading a favorite book, coloring, or going for a walk in nature, prioritize taking care of yourself. By nourishing your mind, body, and soul, you are giving yourself the love and attention you deserve.

Lastly, always remember that you are worthy and deserving of love, happiness, and success. Your struggles do not define you, but rather, they shape you into a resilient and compassionate individual. Embrace your uniqueness and celebrate your strengths. Believe in yourself, because you are capable of achieving anything you set your mind to.

As you continue practicing age regression meditations, know that each session brings you closer to a place of peace and wellbeing. Keep growing, keep learning, and keep nurturing your inner child. You are on a beautiful journey of self-discovery, and we are here to support you every step of the way.

Sweet dreams, Little's. You are loved, cherished, and deserving of all the happiness in the world.

Additional Resources for Little's and Their Caregivers

In addition to the age regression meditations provided in this book, there are several other resources available that can further support Little's and their caregivers in addressing sleep difficulties, self-esteem struggles, and depression. These resources aim to provide guidance, tools, and a sense of community to help Little's navigate their unique challenges.

Online Communities and Forums: Joining online communities and forums specifically designed for Little's can be a valuable resource. These platforms offer a safe space for Little's to connect with others who understand their experiences. Here, they can share their thoughts, seek advice, and find comfort in knowing they are not alone. Caregivers can also benefit from these communities as they can connect with other caregivers, share insights, and gain support.

Therapy and Counseling: Seeking therapy or counseling can be immensely beneficial for Little's dealing with sleep difficulties, self-esteem struggles, or depression. A qualified therapist can provide personalized guidance and support to help Little's better understand their emotions, develop coping mechanisms, and work towards positive change. Caregivers may also benefit from therapy to gain a deeper understanding of their Little's needs and how to provide effective support.

Books and Resources: There are various books and resources available that provide further guidance on age regression meditations, sleep difficulties, self-esteem, and depression within the Little community. These resources offer practical tips, techniques, and exercises that Little's and their caregivers can implement in their daily lives. They can serve as a source of inspiration, education, and validation for both Little's and their caregivers.

Support Groups: Participating in support groups, either online or in-person, can offer a sense of belonging and understanding. These groups provide a space for Little's and their caregivers to share experiences, exchange advice, and find solace in a community of like-minded individuals. Support groups can also be a great platform to learn from others' experiences and gain insights into different coping strategies.

Websites and Blogs: Numerous websites and blogs cater specifically to the Little community and offer a wealth of information, articles, and resources. These platforms cover a range of topics, including sleep difficulties, self-esteem struggles, and depression. Little's and their caregivers can utilize these websites and blogs to access valuable information, expert advice, and practical tips on managing their unique challenges.

Remember, while these additional resources can be incredibly helpful, it is important to seek professional guidance when necessary. Every Little's journey is unique, and finding the right support system is crucial. By utilizing these resources and engaging with supportive communities, Little's and their caregivers can create a nurturing environment that fosters growth, healing, and happiness.